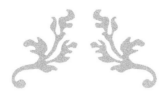

Wood Pellet Smoker And Grill Recipes

The Ultimate Guide To Become A Master At Smoking Meat,
Preparing Marinades And American Barbecue Sauces. Learn The
Best Pork, Beef, And Chicken Recipes

LIAM JONES

Table of Contents

BREAKFAST RECIPES

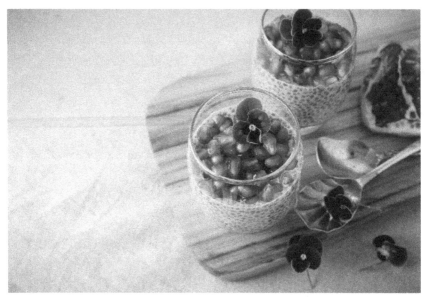

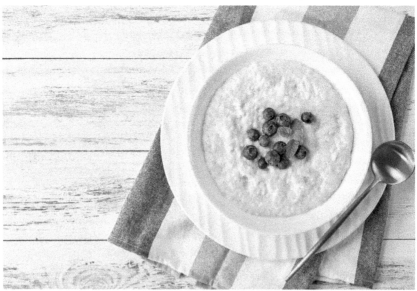

1. *Smoked Apple Pie*

Preparation Time: 15 minutes

Cooking Time: 60 minutes

Servings: 6-8

Ingredients:

- 8 cups cored, peeled, and sliced apples
- 1 tablespoon fresh lemon juice
- ½ cup white sugar
- 2 tablespoons all-purpose flour
- 1 teaspoon ground cinnamon
- ¼ teaspoon ground nutmeg
- A dough of 2 pie crusts (store-bought)
- ¼ cup melted butter
- 1 tablespoon apple cider
- 2 tablespoons heavy whipping cream

Directions:

1. Preheat your smoker to 400-degrees, adding chips to the container. Mix apples, lemon, sugar, flour, cinnamon, and nutmeg in a bowl.
2. Roll out your pie crust into two 11-inch circles. Put one dough circle on a 9-inch pie plate. Brush with melted butter, then add the apple filling.

3. With apple cider, moisten the crust's edges, then cover with the second dough circle. Seal the edges with your fingers.

4. With a knife, make some slits in the top crust and brush with heavy cream. Assuming the smoker is ready now, add the pie and smoke for 50-60 minutes. Cool on a wire rack before serving!

Nutrition: Calories: 529 Protein: 3.1g Carbs: 81g Fat: 23.9g

2. *Orange Bread Pudding*

Preparation Time: 15 minutes

Cooking Time: 1 hour & 40 minutes

Servings: 6-8

Ingredients:

- 8 cups cubed brioche bread
- 3 cups heavy whipping cream
- 2 cups whole milk
- 1 ½ cups white sugar
- Pinch of salt
- Zest of 2 oranges
- 4 eggs
- 2 egg yolks
- 1 teaspoon orange extract

Directions:

1. Preheat your smoker to 230-degrees with the wood chips in the container. In a foil pan, arrange bread cubes in a single layer.
2. When the smoker is ready, add pan and smoke for 40 minutes. While that smokes, put the cream, milk, sugar, and salt in a saucepan.

3. Boil, whisking, to dissolve the sugar. Remove the pan from the hot stovetop. Add orange zest. Put eggs, egg yolks, and orange extract in a bowl and mix.

4. Slowly and carefully whisk in the hot mixture. Add your smoked bread cubes and let them soak for 10 minutes or so on the counter.

5. Grease a smoker-safe skillet and pour in the bread pudding. Smoke for 40 minutes, then check to see if the bread is puffy and golden and the custard has set. Serve warm!

Nutrition: Calories: 533 Protein: 9g Carbs: 59g Fat: 30.9g

3. *Smoky Lemon Bars*

Preparation Time: 15 minutes

Cooking Time: 1 hour & 20 minutes

Servings: 6-8

Ingredients:

- ¾ cup fresh lemon juice
- 1 ½ cups white sugar
- 2 eggs
- 3 egg yolks
- 1 ½ teaspoons cornstarch
- Pinch of salt
- 4 tablespoons cold butter
- ¼ cup olive oil
- ½ tablespoon lemon zest
- 1 ¼ cups flour
- ¼ cup white sugar
- ½ cup powdered sugar
- 1 teaspoon lemon zest
- Pinch of salt
- 10 tablespoons cubed butter
- 3 tablespoons powdered sugar (for serving)

Directions:

1. Preheat your smoker to 350-degrees with wood chips in their container. For now, we're looking at the first list of ingredients.

2. While the smoker heats up, mix lemon juice, sugar, eggs, yolk, cornstarch, and a bit of salt. Pour into a cake pan and smoke for 15 minutes.

3. Stir, then smoke for another 15 minutes. Remove from the smoker. Pour into a saucepan and boil on medium-high.

4. Boil for 60 seconds, then strains into a bowl. Mix in 4 tablespoons butter, oil, and lemon zest.

5. Now for the crust. In a food processor, mix flour, sugar, powdered sugar, lemon zest, and salt. Add in the butter and pulse until you get crumbly dough.

6. Line a 9x9 baking dish using parchment paper and press in the dough. Bake crust for 30 minutes or so until the crust is just turning golden.

7. Pour in the filling and smoke for another 20 minutes. Remove from the smoker and cool to room temperature before sticking in the fridge to chill. Serve with powdered sugar!

Nutrition: Calories: 736 Protein: 6.4g Carbs: 100g Fat: 39.5g

4. *Smoked Ice Cream*

Preparation Time: 15 minutes

Cooking Time: 1 hour & 40 minutes

Servings: 4

Ingredients:

- Ice chips
- Coldwater
- 1-quart heavy cream
- 1 ½ cups heavy cream
- 8 egg yolks
- ¾ cups dark brown sugar
- 1 cup whole milk
- 1 ½ teaspoon pure vanilla extract
- ½ teaspoon of sea salt

Directions:

1. Preheat your smoker to 150-degrees with the chips. Fill a foil pan halfway with ice and then add water, so ice is covered.
2. Put another, smaller foil pan in the ice bath, and pour in 1 quart of cream. Smoke for 1 hour and 40 minutes, stirring.
3. When time is up, put the smoked cream in a container and stick it in the fridge. When it's cooled, mix ½ cup smoked cream with ½ cup fresh cream.

4. Taste and add until you get 2 cups total and the ratio to your liking. Keep leftovers for another use.

5. In a saucepan, mix egg yolks and brown sugar. Add cream mixture and milk, and combine. Heat on medium-low, stirring, until the liquid hits 170-degrees.

6. Pour liquid through a strainer into a container, add vanilla and salt, and put in an ice bath until it hits 45-degrees or lower.

7. When ready, churn according to your ice cream maker's directions. Chill in the freezer for 4-5 hours.

Nutrition: Calories: 434 Protein: 8.5g Carbs: 32g Fat: 30.5g

FISH AND SEAFOOD RECIPES

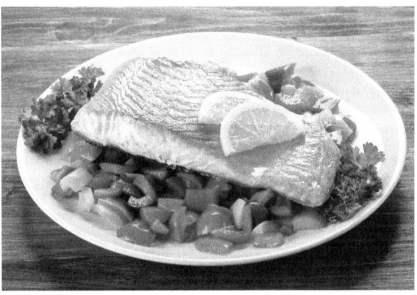

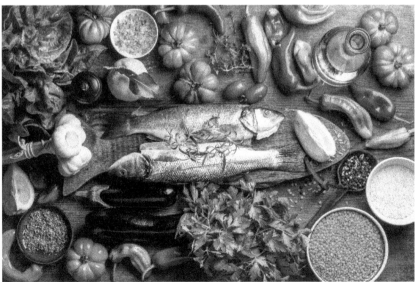

5. *Savory Smoked Trout with Fennel and Black Pepper Rub*

Preparation Time: 15 minutes

Cooking Time: 2 hours 10 minutes

Servings: 10

Ingredients:

- Trout fillet (4,5-lb., 2.3-kg.)

The Rub:

- 2 tbsp. lemon juice
- 3 tbsp. fennel seeds
- 1 ½ tbsp. ground coriander
- 1 tbsp. black pepper
- ½ tsp. chili powder
- 1 tsp. kosher salt
- 1 tsp. garlic powder

The Glaze:

- 3 tbsp. olive oil

The Heat:

- Mesquite wood pellets

Directions:

1. Drizzle lemon juice over the trout fillet and let it rest for approximately 10 minutes.

2. In the meantime, combine the fennel seeds with coriander, black pepper, chili powder, salt, and garlic powder, then mix well.

3. Rub the trout fillet with the spice mixture, then set aside.

4. Plug the wood pellet smoker and place the wood pellet inside the hopper. Turn the switch on.

5. Set the temperature to 225°F (107°C) and prepare the wood pellet smoker for indirect heat. Wait until the wood pellet smoker is ready.

6. Place the seasoned trout fillet in the wood pellet smoker and smoke it for 2 hours.

7. Baste olive oil over the trout fillet and repeat it once every 20 minutes.

8. Once the smoked trout flakes, remove it from the wood pellet smoker and transfer it to a serving dish.

9. Serve and enjoy.

Nutrition: Energy (calories): 185 kcal Protein: 47.32 g Fat: 17.18 g Carbohydrates: 0.94 g

6. *Sweet Smoked Shrimps Garlic Butter*

Preparation Time: 15 minutes

Cooking Time: 20 minutes

Servings: 10

Ingredients:

- Fresh shrimps (2-lbs., 0.9-kg.)

The Rub:

- 2 tbsp. Lemon juice
- ½ tsp. Salt
- ½ tsp. Black pepper

The Glaze:

- 2 tbsp. Butter
- ½ tsp. Garlic powder

The Heat:

- Hickory wood pellets

Directions:

1. Peel the fresh shrimps and drizzle lemon juice over them. Let them rest for several minutes.
2. After that, sprinkle salt and black pepper over the shrimps and spread them in a disposable aluminum pan.
3. Plug the wood pellet smoker and place the wood pellet inside the hopper. Turn the switch on.

4. Set the temperature to 200°F (93°C) and prepare the wood pellet smoker for indirect heat. Wait until the wood pellet smoker is ready.

5. Insert the aluminum pan with shrimps into the wood pellet smoker and smoke the shrimps for approximately 20 minutes.

6. Regularly check the shrimps and once they turn pink, take them out of the wood pellet smoker.

7. Add garlic powder to the butter, then mix until combined. The butter will be soft.

8. Baste the garlic butter over the smoked shrimps and serve.

9. Enjoy!

Nutrition: Amount per 94 g = 1 serving(s) Energy (calories): 99 kcal Protein: 18.6 g Fat: 2.01 g Carbohydrates: 0.21 g

7. *Spiced Smoked Crabs with Lemon Grass*

Preparation Time: 15 minutes

Cooking Time: 20 minutes

Servings: 10

Ingredients:

- Fresh crabs (5-lb., 2.3-kg.)

The Rub:

- 2 tbsp. smoked paprika

- 1 tsp. kosher salt

- 2 tbsp. dried parsley

- 2 tbsp. dried thyme

- 1 tbsp. black pepper

- 1 tsp. cayenne pepper

- 1 tsp. allspice

- ½ tsp. ground ginger

- ½ tsp. cinnamon powder

- 2 lemongrass

The Heat:

- Hickory wood pellets

Directions:

1. Combine the smoked paprika, salt, parsley, thyme, black pepper, ground ginger, cinnamon powder, cayenne pepper, and allspice, then mix well.

2. Arrange the crabs in a disposable aluminum pan, then sprinkle the spice mixture over them.

3. Add lemongrasses on top, then cover the seasoned crabs with aluminum foil.

4. Plug the wood pellet smoker and place the wood pellet inside the hopper. Turn the switch on.

5. Set the temperature to 200°F (93°C) and prepare the wood pellet smoker for indirect heat. Wait until the wood pellet smoker is ready.

6. Insert the aluminum pan with crabs into the wood pellet smoker and smoke the crabs for 30 minutes.

7. Once it is done, take the smoked crabs out of the wood pellet smoker and serve.

8. Enjoy!

Nutrition: Amount per 229 g = 1 serving(s) Energy (calories): 201 kcal Protein: 41.14 g Fat: 2.58 g Carbohydrates: 0.98 g

CHICKEN AND TURKEY RECIPES

8. *Pineapple Teriyaki Turkey Burgers*

Preparation Time: 5 Minutes

Cooking Time: 9 Minutes

Servings: 4

Ingredients:

- 1 tsp. BBQ rub
- 1 can sliced pineapple
- 4 slices Swiss cheese
- 1 cup fresh raw spinach, stems removed
- 4 sets of hamburger buns

Patties:

- 1 lb. ground turkey
- ½ cup bread crumbs
- ¼ cup teriyaki sauce
- 1 small yellow onion, diced
- 2 Tbsp. finely chopped parsley
- 2 cloves garlic, minced
- 1 egg, beaten

Directions:

1. In a large mixing bowl, combine all patty ingredients and mix thoroughly by hand.

2. Divide mixture into four equal parts. Form the four portions into patties and lay them on parchment paper. Sprinkle each patty evenly with BBQ rub. Place in refrigerator for 30 minutes.

3. Bring the pellet grill to high heat. When the pellet grill is hot, place the burgers and pineapple slices. Cook for 4 minutes without flipping. Remove the burgers and cover to keep warm.

4. After burgers are flipped over, add a slice of Swiss cheese to each patty and allow it to melt as the patty finishes cooking. Remove from the pellet grill.

5. Layer burgers on buns with spinach and pineapple.

Nutrition: Calories: 554; Fat: 11g; Protein:26g; Fiber:2g

9. *Juicy Beer Can Turkey*

Preparation Time: 20 Minutes

Cooking Time: 6 hours

Servings: 6-8

Ingredients:

- For the rub
- 4 garlic cloves, minced
- 2 teaspoons dry ground mustard
- 2 teaspoons smoked paprika
- 2 teaspoons salt
- 2 teaspoons freshly ground black pepper
- 1 teaspoon ground cumin
- 1 teaspoon ground turmeric
- 1 teaspoon onion powder
- ½ teaspoon sugar
- For the turkey
- (10-pound) fresh whole turkey, neck, giblets, and gizzard removed and discarded
- tablespoons olive oil
- 1 large, wide (24-ounce) can of beer, such as Foster's
- 4 dried bay leaves
- 2 teaspoons ground sage

- 2 teaspoons dried thyme
- ¼ cup (½ stick) unsalted butter, melted

Directions:

1. To make the rub
2. Following the manufacturer's specific start-up procedure, preheat the smoker to 250°F, and add cherry, peach, or apricot wood.
3. In a small bowl, stir together the garlic, mustard, paprika, salt, pepper, cumin, turmeric, onion powder, and sugar.
4. To make the turkey
5. Rub the turkey inside and out with olive oil.
6. Apply the spice rub all over the turkey.
7. Pour out or drink 12 ounces of the beer.
8. Using a can opener, remove the entire top of the beer can.
9. Add the bay leaves, sage, and thyme to the beer.
10. Place the can of beer upright on the smoker grate. Carefully fit the turkey over it until the entire can is inside the cavity and the bird stands by itself. Prop the legs forward to aid instability.
11. Smoke the turkey for 6 hours, basting with the butter every other hour.
12. Remove the turkey from the heat when the skin is browned and the internal temperature registers 165°F. Remove the

beer can very carefully—it will be slippery, and the liquid inside extremely hot. Discard the liquid, and recycle the can.

13. Let the turkey rest for 20 minutes before carving.

Nutrition: Calories: 300 Cal Fat: 12g Carbohydrates: 1g Fiber: 0g Protein: 42g

10. *Buttered Thanksgiving Turkey*

Preparation Time: 25 minutes

Cooking Time: 5 or 6 hours

Servings: 12 to 14

Ingredients:

- 1 whole turkey (make sure the turkey is not pre-brined)
- 2 batches garlic butter injectable
- 3 tablespoons olive oil
- 1 batch chicken rub
- 2 tablespoons butter

Directions:

1. Supply your smoker with Wood pellets and follow the manufacturer's specific start-up procedure. Preheat the grill, with the lid closed, to 180°F.
2. Inject the turkey throughout with the garlic butter injectable. Coat the turkey with olive oil and season it with the rub. Using your hands, work the rub into the meat and skin.
3. Place the turkey directly on the grill grate and smoke for 3 or 4 hours (for an 8- to 12-pound turkey, cook for 3 hours; for a turkey over 12 pounds, cook for 4 hours), basting it with butter every hour.
4. Increase the grill's temperature to 375°F and continue to cook until the turkey's internal temperature reaches 170°F.

5. Remove the turkey from the grill and let it rest for 10 minutes, before carving and serving.

Nutrition: Calories: 97cal Fat: 4 g Protein: 13 g Carbohydrates: 1 g Fiber: 0 g

11. *Wood pellet simple Smoked Turkey*

Preparation Time: 1 day and 1 hour

Cooking Time: 4 hours and 30 minutes

Servings: 6

Ingredients:

- 2 gallons of water, divided
- 2 cups of sugar
- 2 cups salt
- Ice cubes
- 1 whole turkey
- ½ cup kosher salt
- ½ cup black pepper
- 3 sticks butter, sliced

Directions:

1. Add one quart of water to a pot over medium heat.
2. Stir in the 2 cups each of sugar and salt.
3. Bring to a boil.
4. Remove from heat and let cool.
5. Add ice and the remaining water.
6. Stir to cool.
7. Add the turkey to the brine.
8. Cover and refrigerate for 24 hours.

9. Rinse the turkey and dry with paper towels.

10. Season with salt and pepper.

11. Preheat the Wood pellet grill to 180 degrees F for 15 minutes while the lid is closed.

12. Smoke the turkey for 2 hours.

13. Increase temperature to 225 degrees. Smoke for another 1 hour.

14. Increase temperature to 325 degrees. Smoke for 30 minutes.

15. Place the turkey on top of a foil sheet.

16. Add butter on top of the turkey.

17. Cover the turkey with foil.

18. Reduce temperature to 165 degrees F.

19. Cook on the grill for 1 hour.

Nutrition: Calories: 48.2 Fats: 1.4 g Cholesterol: 21.5 mg Carbohydrates: 0 g Fiber: 0 g Sugar: 0 g Protein: 8.3 g

12. Maple Turkey Breast

Preparation Time: 4 hours and 30 minutes

Cooking Time: 2 hours

Servings: 4

Ingredients:

- 3 tablespoons olive oil
- 3 tablespoons dark brown sugar
- 3 tablespoons garlic, minced
- 2 tablespoons Cajun seasoning
- 2 tablespoons Worcestershire sauce
- 6 lb. turkey breast fillets

Directions:

1. Combine olive oil, sugar, garlic, Cajun seasoning, and Worcestershire sauce in a bowl.
2. Soak the turkey breast fillets in the marinade.
3. Cover and marinate for 4 hours.
4. Grill the turkey at 180 degrees F for 2 hours.
5. Serving Suggestion: Let rest for 15 minutes before serving.
6. Preparation / Cooking Tips: You can also sprinkle dry rub on the turkey before grilling.

Nutrition: Calories: 416 Cal Fat: 13.3 g Carbs: 0 g Protein: 69.8 g Fiber: 0 g

13. *Tandoori Chicken Wings*

Preparation Time: 20 minutes

Cooking Time: 1 hour 20 minutes

Servings: 4-6

Ingredients:

- ¼ Cup Yogurt
- 1 Whole Scallion, minced
- 1 Tablespoon minced cilantro leaves
- 2 teaspoon ginger, minced
- 1 Teaspoon Masala
- 1 teaspoon salt
- 1 teaspoon ground black pepper
- 1 ½ pound chicken wings
- ¼ cup yogurt
- 2 tablespoon mayonnaise
- 2 tablespoon Cucumber
- 2 teaspoon lemon juice
- ½ teaspoon cumin
- ½ teaspoon salt
- 1/8 cayenne pepper

Directions:

1. Combine yogurt, scallion, ginger, garam masala, salt, cilantro, and pepper ingredients in the jar of a blender and process until smooth.
2. Put chicken and massage the bag to cat all the wings
3. Refrigerate for 4 to 8 hours. Remove the excess marinade from the wings; discard the marinade
4. Set the temperature to 350F and preheat, lid closed, for 10 to 15 minutes. Brush and oil the grill grate
5. Arrange the wings on the grill. Cook for 45 to 50 minutes, or until the skin is brown and crisp and meat is no longer pink at the bone. Turn once or twice during cooking to prevent the wings from sticking to the grill.
6. Meanwhile, combine all sauce ingredients; set aside, and refrigerate until ready to serve.
7. When wings are cooked through, transfer to a plate or platter. Serve with yogurt sauce

Nutrition: Calories 241kcal Carbohydrates 11g Protein 12g Fat 16g Saturated Fat 3g

14. *Smoke Roasted Chicken*

Preparation Time: 20 minutes

Cooking Time: 1 hour 20 minutes

Servings: 4-6

Ingredients:

- 8 tablespoon butter, room temperature
- 1 clove garlic, minced
- 1 scallion, minced
- 2 tablespoon fresh herbs such as thyme, rosemary, sage, or parsley
- As needed Chicken rub
- Lemon juice
- As needed vegetable oil

Directions:

1. In a small cooking bowl, mix the scallions, garlic, butter, minced fresh herbs, 1-1/2 teaspoon of the rub, and lemon juice. Mix with a spoon.
2. Remove any giblets from the cavity of the chicken. Wash the chicken inside and out with cold running water. Dry thoroughly with paper towels.
3. Sprinkle a generous amount of Chicken Rub inside the cavity of the chicken.

4. Gently loosen the skin around the chicken breast and slide in a few tablespoons of the herb butter under the skin and cover.

5. Cover the outside with the remaining herb butter.

6. Insert the chicken wings behind the back. Tie both legs together with a butcher's string.

7. Powder the outside of the chicken with more Chicken Rub then insert sprigs of fresh herbs inside the cavity of the chicken.

8. Set temperature to High and preheat, lid closed for 15 minutes.

9. Oil the grill with vegetable oil. Move the chicken on the grill grate, breast-side up then close the lid.

10. After the chicken has cooked for 1 hour, lift the lid. If chicken is browning too quickly, cover the breast and legs with aluminum foil.

11. Close the lid then continue to roast the chicken until an instant-read meat thermometer inserted into the thickest part registers a temperature of 165F

12. Take off the chicken from the grill and let rest for 5 minutes. Serve, Enjoy!

Nutrition: Calories 222kcal Carbohydrates 11g Protein 29g Fat 4g Cholesterol 62mg Sodium 616mg Potassium 620mg

15. *Grilled Asian Chicken Burgers*

Preparation Time: 5 minutes

Cooking Time: 50 minutes

Servings: 4-6

Ingredients:

- Pound chicken, ground
- 1 cup panko breadcrumbs
- 1 cup parmesan cheese
- 1 small jalapeno, diced
- 2 whole scallions, minced
- 2 garlic clove
- ¼ cup minced cilantro leaves
- 2 tablespoon mayonnaise
- 2 tablespoon chili sauce
- 1 tablespoon soy sauce
- 1 tablespoon ginger, minced
- 2 teaspoon lemon juice
- 2 teaspoon lemon zest
- 1 teaspoon salt
- 1 teaspoon ground black pepper
- 8 hamburger buns
- 1 tomato, sliced

- Arugula, fresh
- 1 red onion sliced

Directions:

1. Align a rimmed baking sheet with aluminum foil then spray with nonstick cooking spray.

2. In a large bowl, combine the chicken, jalapeno, scallion, garlic, cilantro, panko, Parmesan, chili sauce, soy sauce ginger, mayonnaise, lemon juice, and zest, and salt and pepper.

3. Work the mixture with your fingers until the ingredients are well combined. If the mixture looks too wet to form patties and add additional more panko.

4. Wash your hands under cold running water, form the meat into 8 patties, each about an inch larger than the buns and ¾" thick. Use your thumbs or a tablespoon, make a wide, shallow depression in the top of each

5. Put them on the prepared baking sheet. Spray the tops with nonstick cooking spray. If not cooking right away, cover with plastic wrap and refrigerate.

6. Set the wood pellet grill to 350F then preheat for 15 minutes, lid closed.

7. Order the burgers, depression-side down, on the grill grate. Remove and discard the foil on the baking sheet so you'll have an uncontaminated surface to transfer the slider when cooked.

8. Grill the burgers for about 25 to 30 minutes, turning once, or until they release easily from the grill grate when a clean metal spatula is slipped under them. The internal temperature when read on an instant-read meat thermometer should be 160F.

9. Spread mayonnaise and arrange a tomato slice, if desired, and a few arugulas leave on one-half of each bun. Top with a grilled burger and red onions, if using, then replace the top half of the bun. Serve immediately. Enjoy

Nutrition: Calories 329kcal Carbohydrates 10g Protein 21g Fat 23g

16. Grilled Sweet Cajun Wings

Preparation Time: 10 minutes

Cooking Time: 45 minutes

Servings: 4-6

Ingredients:

- 2-pound chicken wings
- As needed Pork and Poultry rub
- Cajun shake

Directions:

1. Coat wings in Sweet rub and Cajun shake.
2. When ready to cook, set the wood pellet grill to 350F and preheat, lid closed for 15 minutes.
3. Cook for 30 minutes until the skin is brown and the center is juicy and an instant-read thermometer reads at least 165F. Serve, Enjoy!

BEEF RECIPES

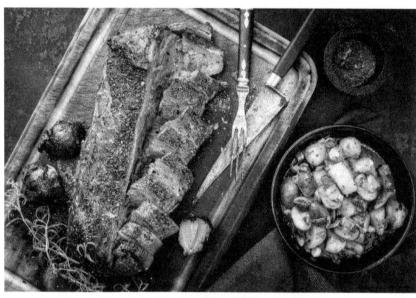

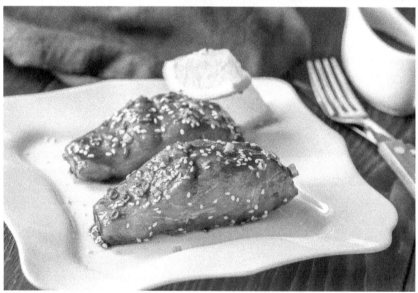

17. *BBQ Brisket*

Preparation Time: 30 minutes

Cooking Time: 6 hours

Servings: 8

Ingredients:

- 1 (12-14) packer beef brisket
- 1 teaspoon cayenne pepper
- 1 teaspoon cumin
- 2 tablespoons paprika
- 1 tablespoon smoked paprika
- 1 tablespoon onion powder
- ½ tablespoon maple sugar
- 2 teaspoon ground black pepper
- 2 teaspoon kosher salt

Directions:

1. Combine all the ingredients except the brisket in a mixing bowl.
2. Season all sides of the brisket with the seasoning mixture as needed and wrap the brisket in plastic wrap. Refrigerate for 12 hours or more.
3. Unwrap the brisket and let it sit for about 2 hours or until the brisket is at room temperature.

4. Preheat the pellet grill to 225°F with lid close, using mesquite or oak wood pellet.

5. Place the brisket on the grill grate and grill for about 6 hours. Remove the brisket from the grill and wrap it with foil.

6. Return brisket to the grill and cook for about 4 hours or until the brisket's temperature reaches 204°F.

7. Remove the brisket from the grill and let it sit for about 40 minutes to cool.

8. Unwrap the brisket and cut it into slices.

Nutrition: Carbohydrates: 22g | Protein: 28g | Fat: 6g | Sodium: 1213mg Cholesterol: 81mg

18. *Fully Loaded Beef Nachos*

Preparation Time: 10 minutes

Cooking Time: 25 minutes

Servings: 6

Ingredients:

- Ground beef (1-lbs, 0.45-kgs)
- 1 large bag of tortilla chips
- 1 green bell pepper, seeded and diced
- Scallions, sliced – ½ cup
- Red onion, peeled and diced – ½ cup
- Cheddar cheese, shredded – 3 cups
- Sour cream, guacamole, salsa – to serve

Directions:

1. In a cast-iron pan, arrange a double layer of tortilla chips.
2. Scatter over the ground beef, bell pepper, scallions, red onion, and finally the Cheddar cheese.
3. Place the cast-iron pan on the grill and cook for approximately 10 minutes until the cheese has melted completely.
4. Take off the grill and serve with sour cream, guacamole, and salsa on the side.

Nutrition: Calories: 160 Cholesterol: 39 Dietary Fiber: 1 | Protein: 10 | Sodium: 361 Total Carbohydrate: 7 | Total Fat: 10

LAMB RECIPES

19. *Wood Pellet Smoked Pulled Lamb Sliders*

Preparation Time: 10 minutes

Cooking Time: 7 hours

Servings: 7

Ingredients:

- 5 lb. lamb shoulder, boneless
- ½ cup olive oil
- ¼ cup dry rub
- 10 oz spritz
- The Dry Rub
- 1/3 cup kosher salt
- 1/3 cup pepper, ground
- 1-1/3 cup garlic, granulated
- The Spritz
- 4 oz Worcestershire sauce
- 6 oz apple cider vinegar

Directions:

1. Preheat the wood pellet smoker with a water bath to 2500 F.
2. Trim any fat from the lamb then rub with oil and dry rub.

3. Place the lamb on the smoker for 90 minutes then spritz with a spray bottle every 30 minutes until the internal temperature reaches 1650 F.

4. Transfer the lamb shoulder to a foil pan with the remaining spritz liquid and cover tightly with foil.

5. Place back in the smoker and smoke until the internal temperature reaches 2000 F.

6. Remove from the smoker and let rest for 30 minutes before pulling the lamb and serving with slaw, bun, or aioli. Enjoy.

Nutrition: Calories: 339 | Fat: 22g | Carbs: 16g | Protein: 18g

20. *Wood Pellet Smoked Leg of Lamb*

Preparation Time: 15 minutes

Cooking Time: 3 hours

Servings: 6

Ingredients:

- 1 leg lamb, boneless
- 4 garlic cloves, minced
- 2 tbsp salt
- 1 tbsp black pepper, freshly ground
- 2 tbsp oregano
- 1 tbsp thyme
- 2 tbsp olive oil

Directions:

1. Trim any excess fat from the lamb and tie the lamb using twine to form a nice roast.
2. In a mixing bowl, mix garlic, spices, and oil. Rub all over the lamb, wrap with a plastic bag then refrigerate for an hour to marinate.
3. Place the lamb on a smoker set at 2500 F. smoke the lamb for 4 hours or until the internal temperature reaches 1450 F.
4. Remove from the smoker and let rest to cool. Serve and enjoy.

Nutrition: Calories: 350 | Fat: 16g | Carbs: 3g | Protein: 49g

21. *Spicy Chinese Cumin Lamb Skewers*

Preparation Time: 20 minutes

Cooking Time: 6 minutes

Servings: 10

Ingredients:

- 1 lb. lamb shoulder, cut into ½-inch pieces
- 10 skewers
- 2 tbsp ground cumin
- 2 tbsp red pepper flakes
- 1 tbsp salt

Directions:

1. Thread the lamb pieces onto skewers.
2. Preheat the wood pellet grill to medium heat and lightly oil the grill grate.
3. Place the skewers on the grill grate and cook while turning occasionally. Sprinkle cumin, pepper flakes, and salt every time you turn the skewer.
4. Cook for 6 minutes or until nicely browned.
5. Serve and enjoy.

Nutrition: Calories: 77 | Fat: 5g | Carbs: 2g | Protein: 6g

22. Garlic and Rosemary Grilled Lamb Chops

Preparation Time: 10 minutes

Cooking Time: 20 minutes

Servings: 4

Ingredients:

- 2 lb. lamb loin, thick-cut
- 4 garlic cloves, minced
- 1 tbsp rosemary leaves, fresh chopped
- 1 tbsp kosher salt
- ½ tbsp black pepper
- 1 lemon zest
- ¼ cup olive oil

Directions:

1. In a small mixing bowl, mix garlic, lemon zest, oil, salt, and black pepper then pour the mixture over the lamb.
2. Flip the lamb chops to make sure they are evenly coated. Place the chops in the fridge to marinate for an hour.
3. Preheat the wood pellet grill to high heat then sear the lamb for 3 minutes on each side.
4. Reduce the heat and cook the chops for 6 minutes or until the internal temperature reaches 1500 F.
5. Remove the lamb from the grill and wrap it in foil. Let it rest for 5 minutes before serving. Enjoy.

Nutrition: Calories: 171 | Fat: 8g | Carbs: 1g | Protein: 23g

PORK RECIPES

23. Easy Pork Steak

Preparation Time: 15 minutes

Cooking Time: 1 hour 30 minutes

Servings: 4

Ingredients:

- 2 lbs. Pork steak
- 2 tbsp. All-purpose rub
- ½ cup Gold N' Bold Sauce

Directions:

1. Begin by applying an all-purpose rub on both sides of pork steak. Get the pellet grill preheated to 275°F, then place pork steaks over the grill,

2. Cook them for about 30 minutes on one side, then flip to the other side and cook as you keep an eye on the hanging pieces to ensure they don't burn.

3. Check if the internal temperature is at 145°F, add some spice, and drizzle with sauce to enhance flavor.

4. Allow to cool for about 5 minutes, then serve and enjoy.

Nutrition: Amount per 263 g = 1 serving(s) Energy (calories): 629 kcal Protein: 57.76 g Fat: 40.21 g Carbohydrates: 5.16 g

24. Pork Butt

Preparation Time: 10 minutes

Cooking Time: 3 hours 10 minutes

Servings: 10

Ingredients:

- 8 lbs. pork butt
- Salt

Directions:

1. Trim and also score the pork butt, then season with salt and preferred rub.
2. Prepare your Pellet grill, then preheat to 225°F.
3. Cook the pork butt for about 3 hours on both side or until the internal temperature gets to 195°F
4. Allow it to cool for about 5 minutes, then serve and enjoy.

Nutrition: Amount per 363 g = 1 serving(s) Energy (calories): 969 kcal Protein: 90.97 g Fat: 64.19 g Carbohydrates: 0 g

25. *Wood Pellet Pork Tenderloin*

Preparation Time: 7 minutes

Cooking Time: 1 hour 30 minutes

Servings: 5

Ingredients

- 1 Pork tenderloin GMG Pork Rub
- 1 Cup of Teriyaki Sauce

Directions

1. You can use 1 to two pork tenderloins. Generously rub the pork tenderloins with the Green Mountain Pork Rub and let it stand aside for about 4 to 24 hours.

2. Set your Wood pellet smoker grill at 320°F (160°C), and when the grill reaches the temperature you are looking for, place in the tenderloin and baste both the sides with a sweet marinade like the Teriyaki sauce

3. Cook for about one and ¼ hours while turning frequently or until the internal temperature displays at least 165° F.

4. Be careful not to overcook the tenderloin because it may lead to obtaining dry meat.

5. Serve and enjoy your dish!

Nutrition: Amount per 148 g = 1 serving(s) Energy (calories): 181 kcal Protein: 27.16 g Fat: 3.2 g Carbohydrates: 8.97 g

26. Apple Orange Pork loin Roast

Preparation Time: 20 Minutes

Cooking Time: 42 Minutes

Servings: 12 Persons

Ingredients:

- 6 Peppercorns
- 1 5-lb. Pork loin
- ½ cup roast Orange juice
- 1 halved Lemon
- ½ cup Kosher salt
- 1 cup Ice water
- ½ tsp. Fennel seeds
- ¼ cup Brown sugar
- 2 tbsps. Olive oil
- ½ tsp. Pepper flakes
- 3 cloves Garlic
- Pepper and salt
- ½ cup Apple juice
- 2 Bay leaves

For the sauce:

- 1 cup Cognac
- 2 tbsps. Butter

- ½ tsp. Pepper flakes
- 1 cup Sugar
- ½ tsp. Minced garlic
- ½ cup Apple juice
- 1, halved Lemon
- 1, sliced thinly Shallot
- ½ cup Orange juice
- ½ tsp. Fennel seeds
- 1 pint, quartered Fresh figs
- 1 cup Ice water

Directions:

1. In a large enough pot, prepare a mixture of brown sugar, salt, bay leaves, garlic, lemon, peppercorns, pepper flakes, fennel seeds, orange juice, and apple. Heat and simmer to dissolve sugar and salt.

2. Transfer the mixture to a container with ice water and refrigerate.

3. In the cooled brine, add pork roast and submerge. Refrigerate for 8–12 hours.

4. Take out the roast, rinse it, and use paper towels to pat dry.

5. Use olive oil to coat the roast and season with pepper and salt.

6. Prepare your Wood Pellet Smoker-Grill by preheating it to a high temperature as per factory instructions. Close the top lid and leave for 12–18 minutes.

7. Roast the meat on the grilling grate for about 23–26 minutes until the internal temperature reaches 140°F.

8. Remove and allow the meat to cool before slicing.

9. Combine all ingredients for the sauce and heat in butter in a large enough pan. Simmer for about 20–30 minutes to reach the desired thickness. Pour the sauce over the sliced pork roast. Your dish is ready to be served.

Nutrition: Amount per 346 g = 1 serving(s) Energy (calories): 503 kcal Protein: 49.26 g Fat: 21.09 g Carbohydrates: 16.25 g

27. *Pork Bone-in Chops with Rosemary and Thyme*

Preparation Time: 20 Minutes

Cooking Time: 52 Minutes

Servings: 6

Ingredients:

- 2 tbsps. butter
- 4 chops, bone-in pork
- 1 sprig rosemary
- 2 sprigs thyme
- Pork rub

Directions:

1. Prepare your Wood Pellet Smoker-Grill by preheating it to a temperature of about 180°F. Close the top lid and leave for 12–18 minutes.
2. Use pork rub to coat the chops properly.
3. Transfer to the grilling grate and let the chops smoke for about 35–40 minutes. That should bring the internal temperature to 130°F.
4. Remove and set aside the chops so they can cool down.
5. Increase the temperature of the smoker grill to high and let the grilling grate preheat.
6. In a cast-iron pan, combine the herbs, butter, and pork chops.
7. Sear the chops, 3–5 minutes on each side.

8. Remove and let the chips cool for about 8–10 minutes.

9. Your dish is ready to be served.

Nutrition: Amount per 105 g = 1 serving(s) 0Energy (calories): 219 kcal Protein: 26.81 g Fat: 11.58 g

Carbohydrates: 0 g

APPETIZERS AND SIDES

28. *Atomic Buffalo Turds*

Preparation Time: 30-45 minutes

Cooking Time: 1.5 hours to 2 hours

Servings: 6-10

Recommended pellets: Hickory, blend

Ingredients:

- 10 Medium Jalapeno Pepper
- 8 oz regular cream cheese at room temperature
- ¾Cup Monterey Jack and Cheddar Cheese Blend Shred (optional)
- 1 teaspoon smoked paprika
- 1 tsp garlic powder
- 1/2 teaspoon cayenne pepper
- Teaspoon red pepper flakes (optional)
- 20 smoky sausages
- 10 slices bacon, cut in half

Directions:

1. Wear food service gloves when using. Jalapeno peppers are washed vertically and sliced. Carefully remove seeds and veins

using a spoon or paring knife and discard. Place Jalapeno on a grilled vegetable tray and set aside.

2. In a small bowl, mix cream cheese, shredded cheese, paprika, garlic powder, cayenne pepper is used, and red pepper flakes if used, until thoroughly mixed.

3. Mix cream cheese with half of the jalapeno pepper.

4. Place the Little Smokies sausage on half of the filled jalapeno pepper.

5. Wrap half of the thin bacon around half of each jalapeno pepper.

6. Fix the bacon to the sausage with a toothpick so that the pepper does not pierce. Place the ABT on the grill tray or pan.

7. Set the wood pellet smoker grill for indirect cooking and preheat to 250 degrees Fahrenheit using hickory pellets or blends.

8. Suck jalapeno peppers at 250 ° F for about 1.5 to 2 hours until the bacon is cooked and crisp.

9. Remove the ABT from the grill and let it rest for 5 minutes before hors d'oeuvres.

29. Bacon Cheddar Slider

Preparation Time: 30 minutes

Cooking Time: 15 minutes

Servings: 6-10 (1-2 sliders each as an appetizer)

Recommended pellet: Optional

Ingredients:

- 1-pound ground beef (80% lean)
- 1/2 teaspoon of garlic salt
- 1/2 teaspoon salt
- 1/2 teaspoon of garlic
- 1/2 teaspoon onion
- 1/2 teaspoon black pepper
- 6 bacon slices, cut in half
- ½Cup mayonnaise
- 2 teaspoons of creamy wasabi (optional)
- 6 (1 oz) sliced sharp cheddar cheese, cut in half (optional)
- Sliced red onion
- ½Cup sliced kosher dill pickles
- 12 mini pieces of bread sliced horizontally
- Ketchup

Directions:

1. Place ground beef, garlic salt, seasoned salt, garlic powder, onion powder, and black pepper in a medium bowl.

2. Divide the meat mixture into 12 equal parts, shape it into small thin round patties (about 2 ounces each) and save.

3. Cook the bacon on medium heat over medium heat for 5-8 minutes until crunchy. Set aside.

4. To make the sauce, mix the mayonnaise and horseradish in a small bowl if using.

5. Set up a wood pellet smoker grill for direct cooking to use pellet grill accessories. Contact the manufacturer to see if there is a pellet grill accessory that works with the wood pellet smoker grill.

6. Spray a cooking spray on the pellet grill cooking surface for best non-stick results.

7. Preheat wood pellet smoker grill to 350 ° F using selected pellets. The Pellet grill surface should be approximately 400 ° F.

8. Grill the putty for 3-4 minutes each until the internal temperature reaches 160 ° F.

9. If necessary, place a sharp cheddar cheese slice on each patty while the patty is on the pellet grill or after the patty is removed from the pellet grill. Place a small amount of mayonnaise mixture, a slice of red onion, and a hamburger pate in the lower half of each roll. Pickled slices, bacon, and ketchup.

30. Grilled Mushroom Skewers

Preparation Time: 5 Minutes

Cooking Time: 60 Minutes

Servings: 6

Ingredients:

- 16 - oz 1 lb. Baby Portobello Mushrooms

For the marinade:

- ¼ - cup olive oil
- ¼ - cup lemon juice
- A small handful of parsley
- 1 - tsp sugar
- 1 - tsp salt
- ¼ - tsp pepper
- ¼ - tsp cayenne pepper
- 1 to 2 - garlic cloves
- 1 - Tbsp balsamic vinegar

What you will need:

- 10 - inch bamboo/wood skewers

Directions:

1. Add the beans to the plate of a lipped container, in an even layer. Shower the softened spread uniformly out ludicrous,

and utilizing a couple of tongs tenderly hurl the beans with the margarine until all around covered.

2. Season the beans uniformly, and generously, with salt and pepper.

3. Preheat the smoker to 275 degrees. Include the beans, and smoke 3-4 hours, hurling them like clockwork or until delicate wilted, and marginally seared in spots.

4. Spot 10 medium sticks into a heating dish and spread with water. It's critical to douse the sticks for in any event 15 minutes (more is better) or they will consume too rapidly on the flame broil.

5. Spot the majority of the marinade fixings in a nourishment processor and heartbeat a few times until marinade is almost smooth.

6. Flush your mushrooms and pat dry. Cut each mushroom down the middle, so each piece has half of the mushroom stem.

7. Spot the mushroom parts into an enormous gallon-size Ziploc sack, or a medium bowl and pour in the marinade. Shake the pack until the majority of the mushrooms are equally covered in marinade. Refrigerate and marinate for 30mins to 45mins.

8. Preheat your barbecue about 300F

9. Stick the mushrooms cozily onto the bamboo/wooden sticks that have been dousing (no compelling reason to dry the

sticks). Piercing the mushrooms was a bit irritating from the outset until I got the hang of things.

10. I've discovered that it's least demanding to stick them by bending them onto the stick. If you simply drive the stick through, it might make the mushroom break.

11. Spot the pierced mushrooms on the hot barbecue for around 3mins for every side, causing sure the mushrooms don't consume the flame broil. The mushrooms are done when they are delicate; as mushrooms ought to be Remove from the barbecue. Spread with foil to keep them warm until prepared to serve

Nutrition: Calories: 230 Carbs: 10g Fat: 20g Protein: 5g

31. Caprese Tomato Salad

Preparation Time: 5 Minutes

Cooking Time: 60 Minutes

Servings: 4

Ingredients:

- 3 - cups halved multicolored cherry tomatoes
- 1/8 - teaspoon kosher salt
- ½ - cup fresh basil leaves
- 1 - tablespoon extra-virgin olive oil
- 1 - tablespoon balsamic vinegar
- ½ - teaspoon black pepper
- ¼ - teaspoon kosher salt
- 1 - ounce diced fresh mozzarella cheese (about 1/3 cup)

Directions:

1. Join tomatoes and 1/8 tsp. legitimate salt in an enormous bowl. Let represent 5mins. Include basil leaves, olive oil, balsamic vinegar, pepper, 1/4 tsp. fit salt, and mozzarella; toss.

Nutrition: Calories 80 Fat 5.8g Protein 2g Carb 5g Sugars 4g

32. Watermelon-Cucumber Salad

Preparation Time: 12 Minutes

Cooking Time: 0 Minutes

Servings: 4

Ingredients:

- 1 - tablespoon olive oil
- 2 - teaspoons fresh lemon juice
- ¼ - teaspoon salt
- 2 - cups cubed seedless watermelon
- 1 - cup thinly sliced English cucumber
- ¼ - cup thinly vertically sliced red onion
- 1 - tablespoon thinly sliced fresh basil

Directions:

1. Consolidate oil, squeeze, and salt in a huge bowl, mixing great. Include watermelon, cucumber, and onion; toss well to coat. Sprinkle plate of mixed greens equally with basil.

Nutrition: Calories 60 Fat 3.5g Protein 0.8g Carb 7.6g

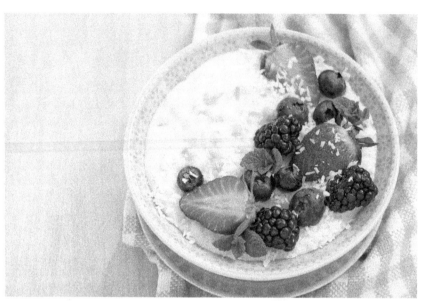

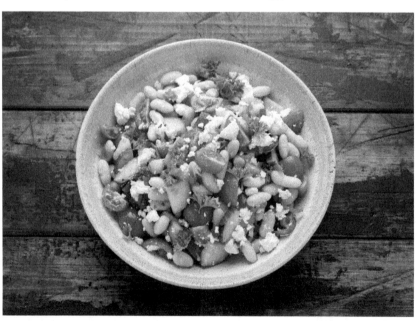

33. *Roasted Spicy Tomatoes*

Preparation Time: 30 Minutes

Cooking Time: 1 Hour and 30 Minutes

Servings: 4

Ingredients:

- 2 lb. large tomatoes, sliced in half
- Olive oil
- 2 tablespoons garlic, chopped
- 3 tablespoons parsley, chopped
- Salt and pepper to taste
- Hot pepper sauce

Directions:

1. Set the temperature to 400 degrees F.
2. Preheat it for 15 minutes while the lid is closed.
3. Add tomatoes to a baking pan.
4. Drizzle with oil and sprinkle with garlic, parsley, salt, and pepper.
5. Roast for 1 hour and 30 minutes.
6. Drizzle with hot pepper sauce and serve.

Nutrition: Calories 118 Total fat 7.6g Total carbs 10.8g Protein 5.4g Sugars 3.7g

Fiber 2.5g, Sodium 3500mg Potassium 536mg

34. Grilled Corn with Honey and Butter

Preparation Time: 30 Minutes

Cooking Time: 10 Minutes

Servings: 4

Ingredients:

- 6 pieces corn
- 2 tablespoons olive oil
- 1/2 cup butter
- 1/2 cup honey
- 1 tablespoon smoked salt
- Pepper to taste

Directions:

1. Preheat the wood pellet grill too high for 15 minutes while the lid is closed.
2. Brush the corn with oil and butter.
3. Grill the corn for 10 minutes, turning from time to time.
4. Mix honey and butter.
5. Brush corn with this mixture and sprinkle with smoked salt and pepper.

Nutrition: Calories 118 Total fat 7.6g Total carbs 10.8g Protein 5.4g Sugars 3.7g Fiber 2.5g, Sodium 3500mg Potassium 536mg

35. Roasted Veggies and Hummus

Preparation Time: 30 Minutes

Cooking Time: 20 Minutes

Servings: 4

Ingredients:

- 1 white onion, sliced into wedges
- 2 cups butternut squash
- 2 cups cauliflower, sliced into florets
- 1 cup mushroom buttons
- Olive oil
- Salt and pepper to taste
- Hummus

Directions:

1. Set the Wood pellet grill too high.
2. Preheat it for 10 minutes while the lid is closed.
3. Add the veggies to a baking pan.
4. Roast for 20 minutes.
5. Serve roasted veggies with hummus.

Nutrition: Calories 118 Total fat 7.6g Total carbs 10.8g Protein 5.4g Sugars 3.7g Fiber 2.5g, Sodium 3500mg Potassium 536mg

36. Grilled Spicy Sweet Potatoes

Preparation Time: 10 minutes

Cooking Time: 35 minutes

Servings: 6

Ingredients:

- 2 lb. sweet potatoes, cut into chunks
- 1 red onion, chopped
- 2 tbsp. oil
- 2 tbsp. orange juice
- 1 tbsp. roasted cinnamon
- 1 tbsp. salt
- ¼ tbsp. Chipotle chili pepper

Intolerances:

- Gluten-Free
- Egg-Free
- Lactose-Free

Directions:

1. Preheat the wood pellet grill to 425°F with the lid closed.
2. Toss the sweet potatoes with onion, oil, and juice.
3. In a mixing bowl, mix cinnamon, salt, and pepper, then sprinkle the mixture over the sweet potatoes.
4. Spread the potatoes on a lined baking dish in a single layer.

5. Place the baking dish in the grill and grill for 30 minutes or until the sweet potatoes are tender.

6. Serve and enjoy.

Nutrition: Amount per 166 g= 1 serving(s) Energy (calories): 109 kcal Protein: 3.86 g Fat: 5.33 g Carbohydrates: 15.01 g

GAME AND ORIGINAL RECIPES

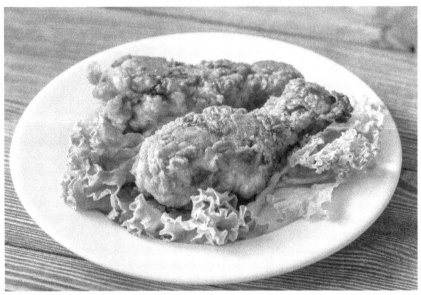

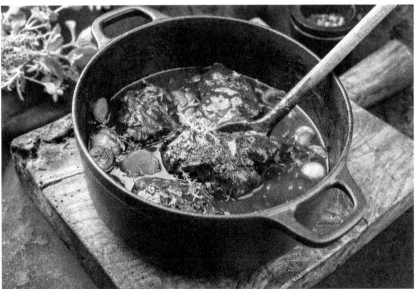

37. *Wood Pellet Elk Jerky*

Preparation Time: 10 minutes

Cooking Time: 6 hours

Servings: 10

Ingredients

- 4 Pounds of elk hamburger
- ¼ Cup of soy sauce
- ¼ Cup of Teriyaki sauce
- ¼ Cup of Worcestershire sauce
- 1 Tablespoon of paprika
- 1 Tablespoon of chili powder
- 1 Tablespoon of crushed red pepper
- 3 Tablespoons of hot sauce
- 1 Tablespoon of pepper
- 1 Tablespoon of garlic powder
- 1 Tablespoon of onion salt
- 1 Tablespoon of salt

Directions:

1. Start by mixing all of the ingredients and seasoning and the elk hamburger in a large bowl; then let sit in the refrigerator for about 12 hours

2. Light your wood pellet smoker to a low temperature of about 160°F

3. Take the elk meat out of your refrigerator and start making strips of the meat manually or with a rolling pin

4. Add smoker wood chips to your wood pellet smoker grill and rub some quantity of olive oil over the smoker grate; layout the strips in one row

5. Warm a dehydrator up about halfway during the smoking process

6. Remove the elk jerky meat off your smoker at about 3 hours

7. Line it into the kitchen.

8. Line your dehydrator with the elk jerky meat and keep it in for about 5 to 6 additional hours

9. Serve and enjoy!

Nutrition: Amount per 37 g = 1 serving(s) Energy (calories): 41 kcal Protein: 1.39 g Fat: 1.39 g Carbohydrates: 6.23 g

38. *Citrus Herb Salt*

Preparation Time: 15 minutes

Cooking Time: 180minutes

Servings: 4

Ingredients:

- 1 C high to quality, coarse kosher salt
- 2 tsp. rosemary
- 2 tsp. thyme
- 2 tsp. granulated garlic
- 2 Limes to zested
- 1 Lemon zested

Directions:

1. Start with a high to quality salt. Don't modest out and get the iodized salt—you genuinely need a decent, coarse salt for this.
2. Include all herbs. Over a different bowl, pizzazz the lemon and two limes (zesting the citrus over the salt blend could add an excessive amount of fluid to the condition).
3. Add the pizzazz to the salt and herb blend, blend well, and store in dashing to the top pack.
4. For a principal couple of days, shake up the pack once every day to guarantee every one of the fixings persuades an opportunity to be dried out by the salt.

5. That will permit the salt to ingest every one of the kinds of herbs and pizzazz. Use varying.

Nutrition: Amount per 109 g = 1 serving(s) Energy (calories): 11 kcal Protein: 0.26 g Fat: 0.08 g Carbohydrates: 3.31 g

39. *Char Siu Baby Back Ribs*

Preparation Time: 120 minutes

Cooking Time: 60minutes

Servings: 6

Ingredients:

Marinade

- 1/3 c hoisin sauce
- 1/3 c soy sauce
- 2 Tbsps. mirin
- 2 Tbsps. honey
- 2 Tbsps. light brown sugar
- 1 Tbsp. Sambal Chili Paste
- 1/2 tbsp. Sesame Oil
- 1/2 Tbsp. Chili Oil
- 1/2 tsp. Chinese 5 spice seasoning
- 3/4 tsp. red food coloring
- Three cloves garlic, minced fine

Basting Liquid

- 1/4 c hoisin
- 1/4 c soy sauce
- 3 Tbsp. honey
- 1 Tbsp. sesame oil

- 1 Tbsp. mirin
- 1 tsp. red miso paste
- 1 tsp. sambal chili paste
- Garnish
- Toasted Sesame Seeds
- Scallions

Directions:

1. Combine all marinade fixings, and race to join.
2. Slice child back ribs into two bone areas. That builds the surface territory for the marinade to give more flavor
3. Spot ribs and marinade in a hurdle to top back, evacuating however much air as could be expected, and marinate for in any event 4Hrs. Marinate medium-term if conceivable.
4. Evacuate ribs and hold marinade.
5. Spot ribs on smoker at 250F. Try not to contact the principal 2Hrs.

6. Join saved marinade and extra treating fluid fixings into a sauce skillet. Bring to a stew, mixing once in a while, for 10mins. Take out from the heat.

7. At the 2hrs mark, treat ribs with seasoning fluid, and rehash each 30mins, until ribs are delicate, roughly 4Hrs.

8. Cut ribs segments into singular ribs, embellish with sesame seeds and scallions.

Nutrition: Amount per 69 g = 1 serving(s) Energy (calories): 123 kcal Protein: 3.24 g Fat: 5.31 g Carbohydrates: 17.29 g

40. Ancho-Dusted Jícama Sticks with Lime

Preparation Time: 15 minutes

Cooking Time: 30 minutes

Servings: 8

Ingredients:

- 1 2-pound jícama, trimmed and peeled
- 2 tablespoons good-quality olive oil
- 2 teaspoons ancho chile powder
- Salt
- 1 lime, cut into wedges

Directions:

1. Start the coals or heat the gas grill for medium-high direct cooking. Make sure the grates are clean.
2. Cut the jícama into ½-inch slices. Brush the slices on both sides with olive oil. Put the slices on the grill directly over the fire. Close the lid and cook, turning once, until they develop grill marks, 7 to 10 minutes per side.
3. Transfer the jícama to a cutting board and cut the slices into ½-inch-wide sticks. Put on a serving platter and sprinkle with the ancho powder and salt to taste, turning them to coat

evenly. Squeeze the lime wedges over them, again turning to coat evenly, and serve.

Nutrition: Calories: 49 | Fats: 0.1g Cholesterol: 0mg Carbohydrates: 12g | Fiber: 6.4g | Sugars: 0g

Proteins: 1g